STRETCHING MATTERS

SIMPLE WORKOUTS TO KEEP YOU STRETCHED AND END EVERYDAY PAIN

Table of Contents

INTRODUCTION

As we grow old, our bodies get weaker, and thus, we are not able to move as fast as before. Furthermore, the less we move, the more tightly our muscles and joints become. Yet this isn't our normal state—in truth, our bodies were intended for development.

Stretching is a delicate, basic movement that anyone can do. Specialists regularly endorse stretching to patients to alleviate ongoing throbbing painfulness and to improve the scope of mobility and adaptability. People who appreciate a functioning lifestyle find that regular stretching improves athletic execution and decreases the danger of injury.

We realize how significant stretching is. My work as a seasoned yoga instructor, exercise physiologist, and graduate-level health educator has affected a great number of lives, and has made me a leading master in the health and wellness industry. *Stretching Matters* meets you at your present level of stretching capacity. It guides you step-by-step through each stretch, arming you with the confidence to advance into more profound levels of stretching for improved adaptability and quality.

Stretching Matters is your all-in-one guide to creating a stretching routine that is tailor-fit to your specific needs. In these pages you'll find:

❖ Point by point delineations that give visual guides to the right positioning of your body

❖ Straightforward clarifications of the cutting edge looking into each stretch and how it functions

❖ "Switch things up" tips for the modifications that allow you to increase or decrease intensity level while stretching

❖ The most current, state-of-the-art information on the fundamental and appropriate how-to-do stretching

Beginning to end guidance—from planning to self-customization—*Stretching Matters* conveys stretching choices that consider your present issues and the lifestyle you need to lead.

Introduction

Regardless of your age or level of movement, *Stretching Matters* will remove the disarray from starting and put the happiness into stretching.

Sore, stiff, and aching muscles? Stretching is essential for adaptability and muscle care. Be that as it may, odds are, a brisk stretch isn't included in your daily routine. Regardless of whether or not you use up all available time after your exercise, don't feel you have adequate twinges to warrant testing your adaptability, or don't have the skill, squeezing in some TLC is a higher priority than you understand.

CHAPTER 1

THE ADVANTAGES OF DAILY STRETCHING

Stretching before exercise is valuable for preparing the body for exercise and helping to decrease injury. Dynamic stretches (those stretches that involve development) are viewed as superior to static stretches (those that you hold) pre-exercise. Using the scope of-movement is better for warming the body up for exercise. Stretching accompanies the following advantages:

Boosts your versatility

Stretching can improve your scope of development and versatility if rehearsed routinely.

Improves your stance

Stretching can assist with enhancing position. Muscle gatherings, for example, hamstrings and those found around the chest, can get logically tighter by being constrained into a similar situation for a considerable length of time, as is regularly the situation following a day at the work area. Stretching these muscles consistently can assist with counteracting a portion of the impact of those hours spent sitting.

Minimizes injury hazard

Stretching can assist with reducing the danger of injury and alleviate specific injuries (for example, lower back pain), especially if the absence of adaptability is an issue in the surrounding muscles.

Relax

Stretching can be extremely relaxing! Unlike your cardio or quality routine, there is no actual consumption involved with stretching, so it's an ideal time to sit (or lie) back and center around breathing deeply, allowing pressure to scatter, and gather your contemplations for the afternoon.

CHAPTER 2

ATTEMPT THESE DAILY STRETCHES

Go through 5-10 minutes warming up before stretching to increase blood flow to the muscles before you stretch—this could be something as simple as a short walk or taking a couple of flights of stairs.

1. The neck stretch

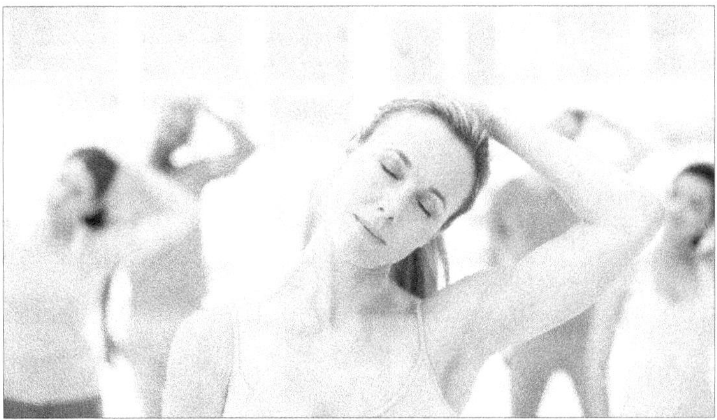

This neck stretch can be performed sitting or standing and is an extraordinary method to ease developed neck pressure from a day at your PC.

✓ **Try this:** From a specific position, place your left hand on the right side of your head and have your right arm behind your back. Gently pull your head to the left side until you feel a delicate stretch in your neck. Hold for 20-30 seconds. Repeat on the opposite side.

2. The standing quad stretch

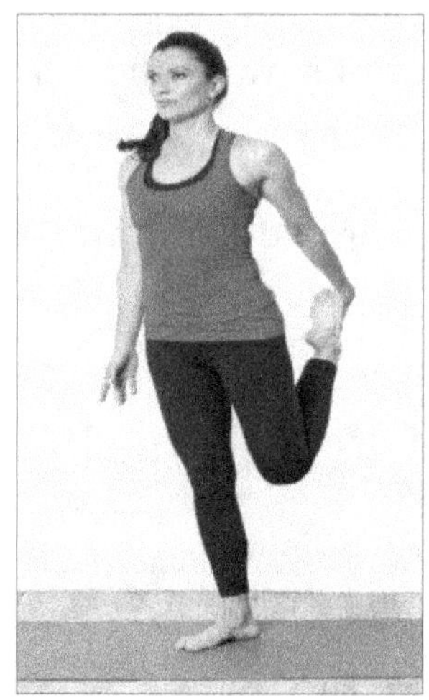

This can assist with easing strain that develops in hip and thigh muscles through the course of the day. Keeping these muscles adaptable may help with keeping both knee and back pain under control.

✓**Attempt this:** From a standing position, using a wall or entryway for help if required, twist your correct leg, snatch the highest point of your right foot towards your right butt cheek, knee pointing down at the floor. You should feel a stretch down in the front of your right thigh. Then, twist the hips forward to feel the stretch at the apex of your thigh. Hold for 20-30 seconds. Change to the left leg.

3. The chest stretch

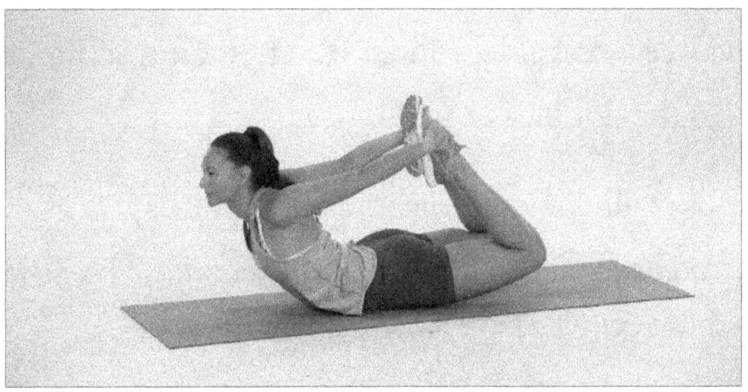

This chest stretch is one of the least demanding approaches to stretching your chest muscles, which can get tight and exhausted if you invest a great deal of energy sitting or on gadgets, and can add to weak stances.

Stand tall and fasten your hands behind your back, squeezing your shoulder bones as you raise your arms. Lift it higher to feel a stronger stretch. Hold for 20-30 seconds.

Stretching toward the end of your exercise can help support your flexibility, lessen the danger of injury, and reduce muscle pressure in your body. It can even improve your presentation whenever you work out.

When you're coming up short on time, stretching can assume a lower priority, and it might be tempting to skip it.

Stretching after an exercise doesn't need to take long, and you can discover accessible routes by stretching a few muscle groups on the double.

This book will look at six straightforward yet profoundly viable stretches you can add to your exercise.

CHAPTER 3

ADVANTAGES OF STRETCHING AFTER AN EXERCISE

The benefits of stretching have been discussed. Here's a rundown of the critical ways that stretching after an exercise can support you.

More noteworthy flexibility and range of movement

Stretching helps to improve the flexibility of your joints: Having more exceptional flexibility allows you to move around more effectively, and it can likewise enhance the range of movement in your joints. The range of movement is how far you can move a joint an ordinary way before it stops.

Better posture and less back pain

Tight, tense muscles can prompt poor posture. At the point when you sit or stand inaccurately, you regularly put additional weight and strain on your muscles. This can prompt back pain and different kinds of musculoskeletal pain.

As per a 2015 study trusted Source, joining a quality preparing routine with stretching activities can assist ease with backing and shoulder pain. It might likewise energize appropriate arrangements, which may help improve your posture.

Stretching your muscles normally may also help existing back injuries and lower your hazard for back injuries later on.

Less muscle pressure and reduced stress

Stress is a part of our normal day-to-day existence. In any case, now and again, it can feel overpowering. Significant levels of stress can make your muscles worry, which can cause you to feel as though you're conveying stress in your body.

Stretching muscles that feel tense and tight can help loosen them up. This may help bring down your stress levels and assist you with feeling more settled.

Improved blood flow

As indicated by a 2018 creature study trusted Source, daily stretching can help improve your blood flow. Expanded blood flow to your muscles can assist them with mending all the more rapidly after an exercise. Better blood flow may likewise help forestall muscle irritation and stiffness after an exercise.

CHAPTER 4

WHAT'S THE DIFFERENCE BETWEEN DYNAMIC AND STATIC STRETCHING?

You may have heard of static and dynamic stretching and consider how they differ.

Static stretching includes stretches that you hold for a while, normally 20 to 60 seconds. You don't move while you're stretching a specific muscle or gathering of muscles.

Static stretching is regularly done toward the end of your exercise when your muscles are warm and loose.

Dynamic stretching again includes dynamic developments. With this sort of a stretch, your joints and muscles experience a full range of movement.

Dynamic stretching is normally done before an exercise to help warm up your muscles and get your pulse up. For example, a sprinter may run or jump to pump their legs up before beginning a race.

Synopsis

Dynamic stretching includes dynamic developments, such as moving your arms or legs through a full range of movement. These stretches are generally done before you start an exercise set.

Static stretching includes stretches that you hold for a while, without development. These stretches are done toward the end of your exercise when your muscles are progressively loose.

CHAPTER 5

EXTRAORDINARY POST-EXERCISE STRETCHES TO ATTEMPT

At the point when you stretch after your exercise, concentrate on the muscles you utilized while you were working out.

You needn't to bother with any gear. However, a yoga mat or other padded surface can diminish the weight on your joints and make your stretches progressively agreeable.

1. Thrusting hip flexor stretch

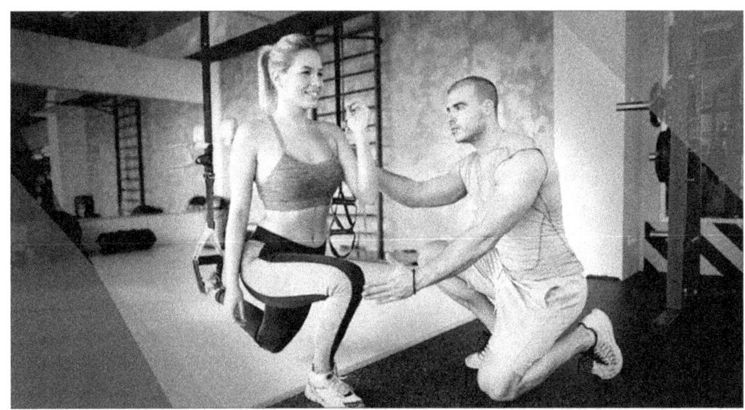

This stretch focuses on the muscles in your hips, quads, and the glutes.

Kneel on your left knee. Keep your correct knee twisted, with your right foot level on the floor before you.

Bend forward and stretch out your left hip toward the floor.

Hold this stretch for 30 to 60 seconds before switching legs and doing the opposite side.

2. Piriformis stretch

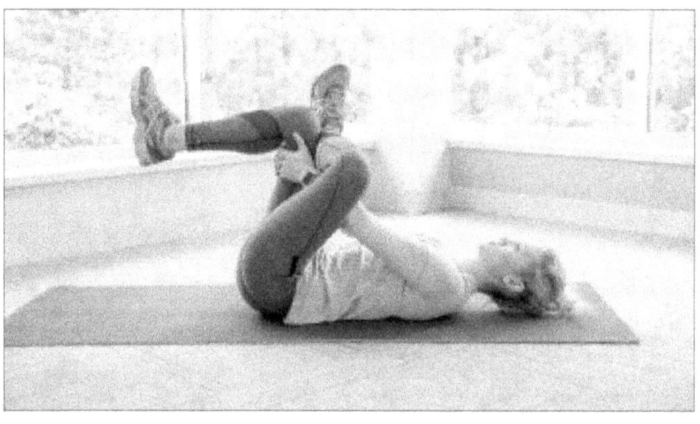

This stretch focuses on your piriformis muscle that runs from the base of your spine to your thigh bone. This muscle can influence how well you move your hips, back, legs, and rear end.

Start by sitting on the floor with your legs stretched out before you.

Keeping your right leg level on the floor, lift your left leg and spot your left lower leg on your right knee.

Marginally curve your back and lean forward until a stretch is felt in your posterior. Hold this stretch for 30 seconds. At that point, repeat with your right leg on your left knee.

Repeat several times with every leg.

3. Cat-cow stretch

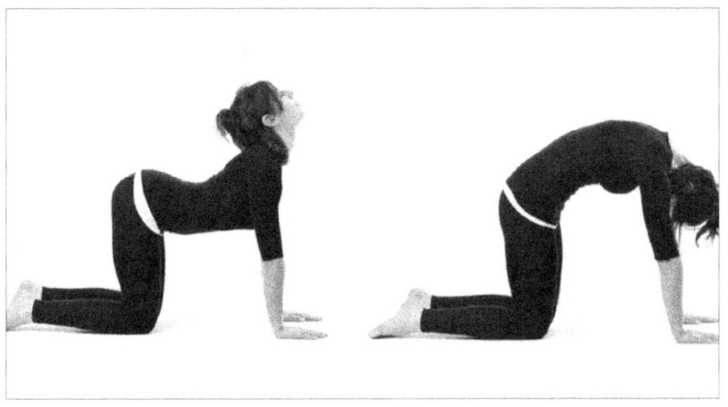

This stretch targets your back muscles.

Start with your knees and hands on the floor with your spine in an unbiased, loosened up arrangement.

Breathe in as you let your stomach sink toward the floor, squeezing your chest forward.

Lift your head, loosen up your shoulders, and start to breathe out.

Round your spine upward, taking care of your tailbone and squeezing your pubic bone forward.

Loosen up your head toward the floor and repeat. Do this multiple times in the range of a moment, if you can.

4. Standing calf stretch

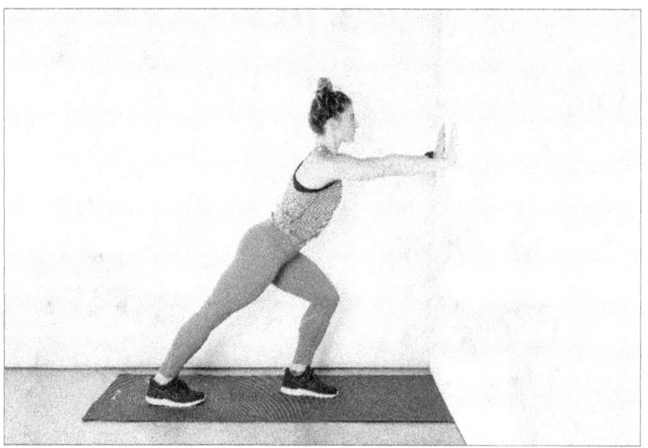

As the name recommends, this stretch targets your lower leg muscles.

Start by remaining close to a seat for help with one foot before the other, front knee marginally bowed.

Keep your back knee straight, your two heels on the floor, and lean forward toward the wall or seat.

You will feel a stretch along the calf of your leg.

Hold this stretch for 20 to 30 seconds.

Switch legs, and do 2 or 3 reiterations on each side.

5. Overhead triceps stretch

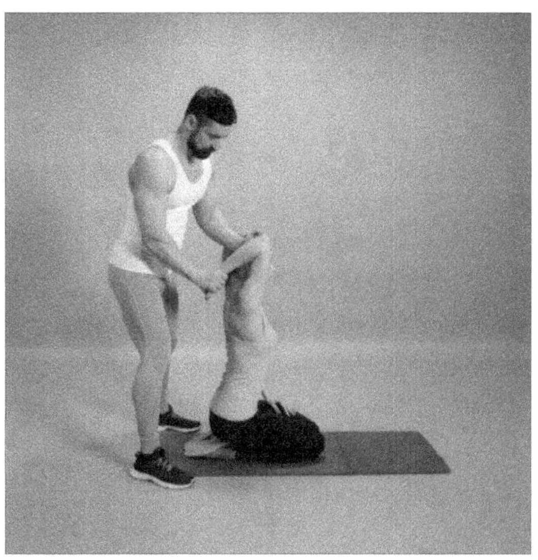

This stretch focuses on your triceps and the muscles in your shoulders.

Remain with your feet hip-width separated and roll your shoulders back and down to discharge any strain.

Lift your right arm up to the roof and twist your elbow to bring your right palm down toward the focal point of your back.

Bring your left hand up to pull your right elbow, descending gently.

Do this for 20 to 30 seconds before exchanging arms.

Repeat on both sides several times, endeavoring to get a more deep stretch with every reiteration.

6. Standing bicep stretch

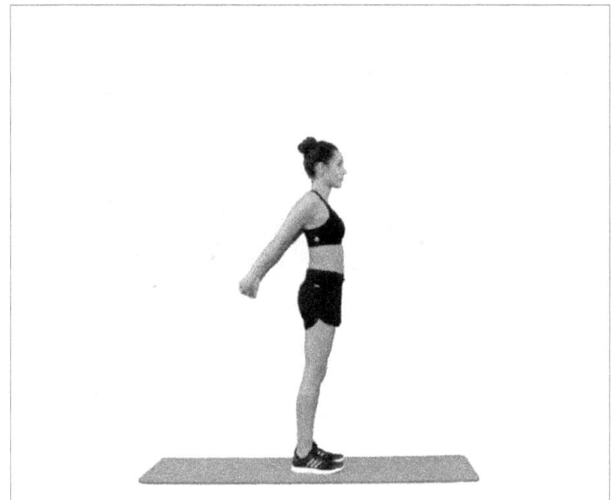

This stretch targets your biceps where they meet the muscles in your chest and shoulders.

Stand upright. Spot your hands behind your back and interweave your hands at the base of your spine.

Fix your arms and turn your hands, so your palms are looking down.

At that point, raise your arms as high as you can until you feel a stretch in your biceps and shoulders.

Do this for 30 to 40 seconds.

Repeat several times.

7. The cat stretch

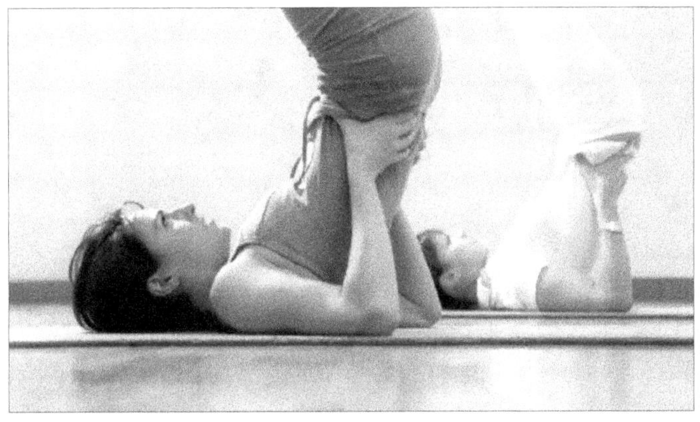

This is an extraordinary minimal stretch to do by the day's end. It's useful for stretching out both upper and lower back and quietly works your center muscle as well.

* Do this: Start in an all-fours sitting position with your back flat before rounding your spine and arching your back and dropping chin to chest. Gently contract your abdominals as you do this, taking care not to hold your breath. Hold for five seconds, unwind and repeat. Do a total of five curves.

8. The hamstring stretch

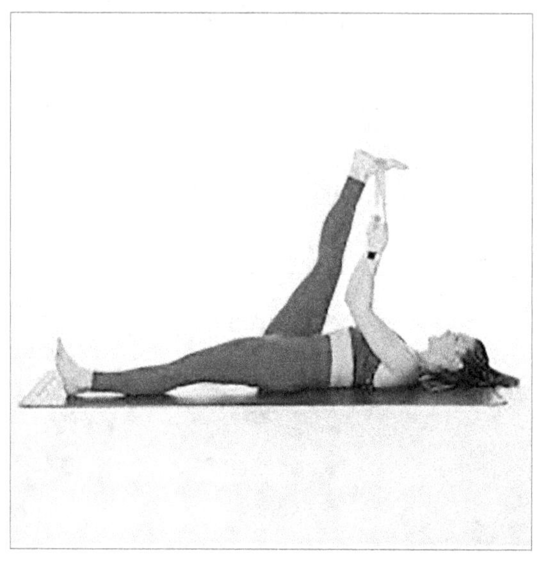

A lying hamstrings stretch is an extraordinary method to stretch out backs of legs and an opportunity to rest simultaneously! Maintaining adaptability in the hamstrings is significant, especially if you're dynamic or potentially deskbound as tight hamstrings can put extra weight on the lower back, aggravating or causing lower back pain.

* Do this: With both of your legs bent, lie on the floor and wrap an obstruction band, scarf or towel around the base of one foot (your other foot ought to remain on the floor). Gradually broaden your leg upwards and to a right angle—

you should feel a stretch but no pain. Hold for 30 seconds before repeating on the opposite side.

9. The bum stretch

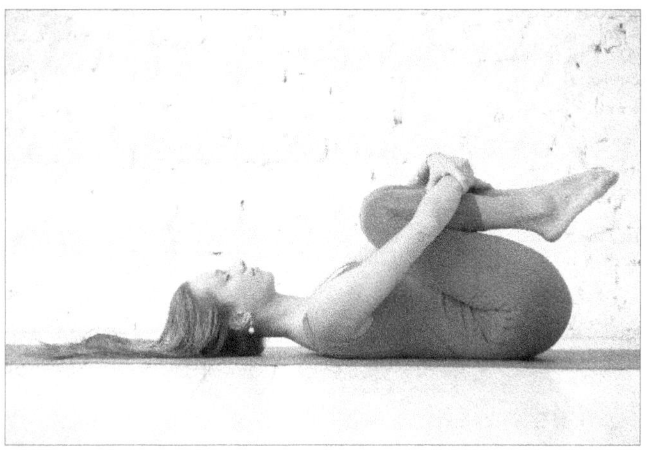

A decent glute (butt cheek) stretch shouldn't be disregarded either—this can likewise assist with easing any hip or lower back stiffness.

* Do this: Lie on your back with both legs bent and feet flat on the floor. Raise your legs off the floor and lift your thigh over the knee of your left leg. Pull your left thigh and push your right foot (keep your right foot straight) towards you until you feel a stretch in your right butt cheek. Hold for 30 seconds. Repeat on the opposite side.

10. The hip stretch

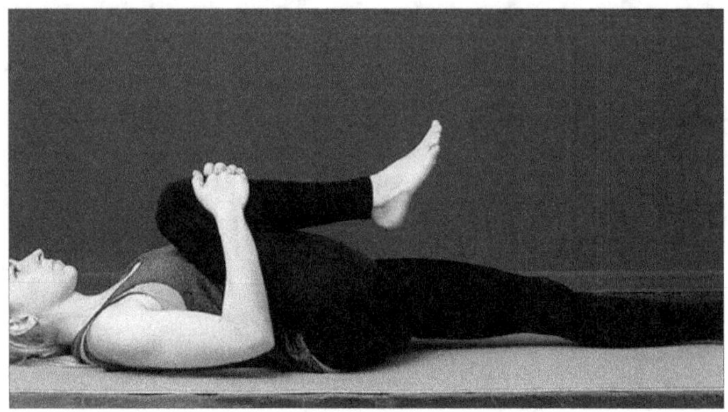

Finish your stretching grouping with the fantastic hip move exercise. Additionally, this versatile hip roll stretches out muscles around your hips, lower back, and chest.

* Do this: Lie on your back with legs bent at the knee and flat feet, arms out to the side. Roll your hips and legs to one side, keeping feet flat on the floor as you move to the left. Hold for 3 seconds before returning to focus and repeating on the opposite side. Play out an aggregate of 10 rolls.

Wellbeing tips

Try not to stretch to the point of pain. You should feel mild pressure as you stretch your muscles. If you feel pain, stop immediately.

Watch your stance. Focus on your posture with each stretch. Keep your jawline up, spine straight, center drawn in, and your shoulders lined up with your hips.

Inhale throughout your stretches. Breathing will assist you with calming pressure and strain in your muscles, and it might also improve the nature of your stretches and assist you with holding a stretch longer.

Start slowly. Try not to attempt to do too much the first time you stretch after an exercise. Start with only a couple of stretches and include more reiterations and stretches as you become accustomed to them.

The main concern

Stretching in the wake of working out can help you receive numerous benefits.

When you stretch your muscles after an exercise, you're helping to kick your body off on recuperation while also discharging pressure and strain, and boosting the flexibility of your joints.

If you're uncertain how to extend securely, ask a certified fitness coach to show you how. If needed, make sure to consult with your health care provider before beginning any new exercise program, particularly if you have a physical issue or an ailment.

Flexibility is one of the five segments of wellness, so stretching ought to be an essential piece of each exercise program. Here are Top 10 Reasons for why you ought to consistently set aside the effort to extend:

1. Diminishes muscle stiffness and expands the range of motion. Stretching improves your range of motion, which may likewise slow the degeneration of your joints.

2. May diminish your risk of injury. An adaptable muscle is less likely to be injured if you need to make an unexpected move. By expanding the range of motion in a specific joint through stretching, you can diminish the obstruction on your body's muscles while engaging in different exercises.

3. Soothes post-exercise a throbbing painfulness. After a laborious exercise, stretching your muscles helps keep them free and decreases the effect that can prompt post-exercise throbbing painfulness.

4. Proving act. Stretching the muscles of the shoulders, lower back, and chest helps keep your back in the better arrangement and improves your stance.

5. Diminishes pressure. Extended muscles hold less strain and can assist you with feeling less pushed.

6. Diminishes strong pressure and enhances solid unwinding. Incessantly tense muscles will, in general, take away their own circulation, bringing about an absence of oxygen and fundamental supplements. Stretching allows your muscles to unwind.

7. Improves mechanical proficiency and generally practical execution. Because an adaptable joint requires less energy to move through a more extensive range of motion, an adaptable body improves performance typically by making more energy-effective developments.

8. Readies the body for the pressure of exercise. Stretching before exercise allows your muscles to slacken up, ready to endure the impact of the action you decide to do.

9. Advances in circulation. Stretching expands blood supply to your muscles and joints, which allows for

more prominent supplement transportation and improves the flow of blood through your whole body.

10. Diminishes the risk of low-back pain. Flexibility in the hamstrings, hip flexors, and muscles appended to the pelvis assuages weight on the lumbar spine, which decreases your risk of low-back pain.

CHAPTER 6

INSTRUCTIONS TO EXERCISE WHEN YOU'RE WORKING (9-5)

If one thing fends a physician off—other than apples, obviously—it's exercise.

Notwithstanding improving one's disposition and shedding those additional pounds, being truly dynamic all the time forestalls and deals with a broad scope of medical issues, including stroke, type 2 diabetes, wretchedness—the rundown continues endlessly.

CHAPTER 7

TIME TABLE FOR PROPER STRETCHING

In any case, I know what you're going to say.

You're spending extended periods of time grinding away, so there's no opportunity to exercise. Children happened, so there's no opportunity to exercise. You're simply so drained from all the side tasks, obligations, even the horrendous climate. There's no opportunity to exercise!

Also, you may very well be correct. By and large, 21% of every waking hour over a 76-year lifespan is spent grinding away, which is a huge lump out of your time.

Be that as it may, stop and think for a minute. The way to add exercise into that tight timetable of yours is to start small.

A study demonstrated that even 15 minutes of light activity can improve your wellbeing and life span. As reported by the Centers for Disease Control and Prevention, a few 10-minute workouts are similarly as compelling as a more extended length workout—as long as they equal 150 minutes of physical movement per week.

So as opposed to changing your timetable unexpectedly, have a go at adding little bits of exercise all through your bustling workday.

Here's how to do that:

1. Start a morning exercise routine

Doing as little as 10-15 minutes of morning exercise can improve your wellbeing and increase your energy for the afternoon.

Starting your day with a bit of exercise is a brilliant method to awaken the body and brain, just as you get the juices streaming. Easy to say if you're a morning individual, correct?

There are different wellbeing and health benefits when practicing in the morning, beginning from the way that your body is in the early hours, the body is in excellent condition for development and muscle development. Your body is asking to be effectively utilized.

Still not convinced? Here are a couple of realities that will prevail upon even the no-nonsense night owls:

Morning exercise supports the metabolic rate. Fundamentally, a morning workout improves your digestion, which suggests that you'll have the option to take more calories all through the remainder of the day.

Practicing in the morning develops consistency. Staying with an exercise plan can be difficult if you have other pressing undertakings on your plate. Doing some exercise in the morning allows for different needs and makes it less likely that you'll avoid your workout totally.

It improves mental and physical energy. Engaging in a morning exercise routine will leave you feeling conscious and it will also renew your energy levels. So if you're attempting to drop those caffeine levels, this is the best approach.

So where to start if you're not used to doing exercise in the morning?

Stretching improves adaptability and awakens the body, making it an extraordinary expansion to the morning exercise routine.

Apply the "start small" standard. There's no compelling reason to drive yourself to work out for 1 hour in a row directly after slithering up – unless that is the thing that you need. It's fine to let yourself start bit by bit. In any event, awakening, say, 10-15 minutes sooner than your standard time of moving around can be a kick-off.

There are a lot of short morning exercise routine models out there. Here are a few thoughts:

❖ Morning stretches. Specialists underscore that stretching in the morning improves pose, relieves agony and throbs in your body, just as builds body stream. Most stretches take a limited quantity of time and require scarcely any space. Regardless of whether you're short on time, getting even a few stretching exercises into your morning routine will bring positive vibes for the remainder of the day. Here are two exercises you ought to do each morning.

❖ Short bodyweight workouts. Doing empowering exercises like jumping jacks or bikes functions as a unique stretch for the body and increases your pulse. Attempt this 7-minute workout or a progressively delicate development routine that will even now get the blood pumping.

❖ Morning yoga. This is an extraordinary choice for the people who need to discover their Zen as well as manage stressful cutoff times. Practicing yoga in the morning helps with keeping a quiet psyche and sets a pace for the afternoon. Do Sun Salutations if possible to improve blood flow and reinforce the body.

2. <u>Move more at work</u>

Practicing during the workday improves profitability.

Many salaried employments today require loads of sitting at your work area and composing endlessly at the PC. This is not a reason to skip exercise when you're grinding away. Research shows that practicing during the workday can help your efficiency.

It appears bosses notice this change as well. It's become a remarkable thing for organizations to establish a devoted health and workout zone in the working environment. Fortunately for those individuals who don't have such brilliant advantages, remaining truly dynamic doesn't generally require extra gear and is more straightforward than you may suspect.

Here are several techniques on how to exercise when you are busy working without attempting excessive workouts:

Take strolling breaks. Change riding the elevator to taking the stairs. Walk to the highest floor of the building, give yourself time to breathe, and stroll back down. Other than informing your partner to, get over here and take a walk. Dump the seat and take a walk because every bit of progression checks out as good.

Challenge your associates. Odds are you're not the only one searching for a chance to add a little exercise to your day to day routine. Discovering similarly invested partners can be very encouraging. Do a day to day challenge of squats, jumps, push-ups, boards, or wall stands where you need to finish the exercise for a set number of reiterations or a specific length. Staying in shape with your peeps will increase the odds of you adhering to the responsibility.

Sit on a fitness ball. When substituting your seat with a fitness ball, your body is continually attempting to adjust itself, in this way helping you practice better stance and driving legitimate spine arrangement. It also fortifies your stomach muscles and helps battle stalling.

Remaining mobile at work doesn't require additional hardware—taking strolling breaks with associates can be fun and persuasive.

Things being what they are, sitting for extended periods is the guilty party of numerous wellbeing concerns. After some time, it debilitates certain parts of your body, particularly in the back and hips. This can cause migraines, back, and hip pain, and at last, make it harder to center and remain healthy.

We have discovered that sitting at a work area can prompt upper cross disorder, where you build up an adjusted upper back and shoulder act, and a forward head position. This postural awkwardness can cause shoulder agony and cerebral pains, among different indications.

Sitting throughout the day can likewise bring about lower cross disorder. At the point when you're sitting, the front of your hips and lower back become tight, while the glutes and abs are debilitated. This unevenness causes the lower back to curve and the pelvis to turn downwards.

Study this graph:

Fortunately, adding the accompanying six stretching exercises into your workday (or after work) will lighten the irritation and support your upper and lower body.

1. Pec stretch – stretches the chest muscles

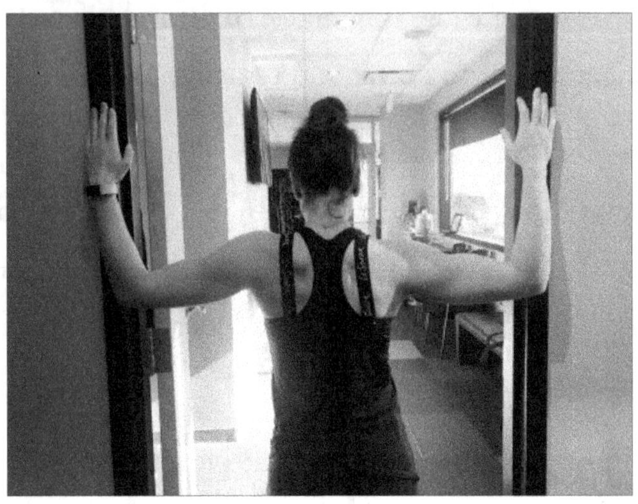

The most efficient technique to do it: place your hands on either side of an entryway; keep your elbows twisted at 90°. Venture forward, extending your arms until you feel a stretch. Hold for 15-30 seconds.

2. Upper trapezius stretch – stretches the upper back

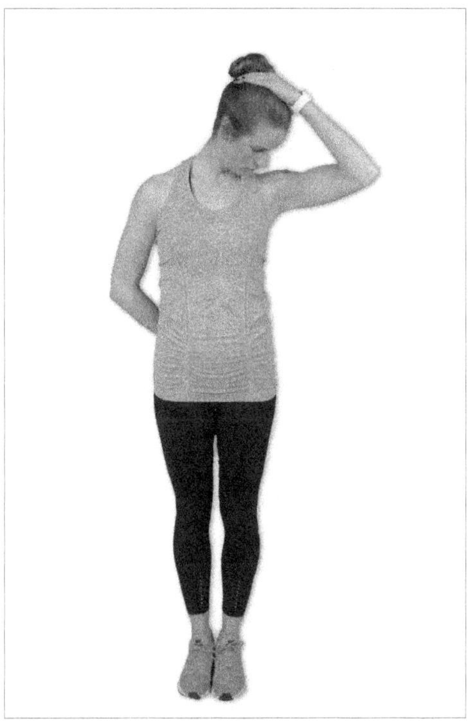

Step by step instructions to do it: place your hand on your head and gently pull down. Keep your contrary shoulder lowered. Hold for 15-30 seconds.

<u>3. Columns – works the rhomboids, which unite your shoulder bones.</u>

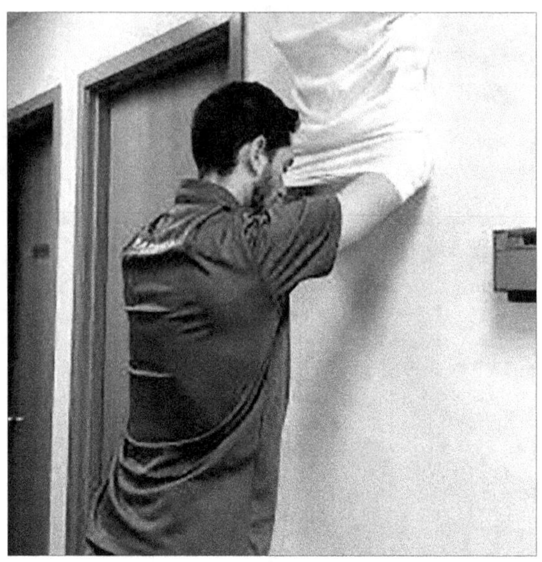

Step by step instructions to do it: you'll need a Thera band for this. Connect it to an entryway, fixing your arms and remaining with your feet shoulder-width separated. Pull the band back to ensure your arms are at a 90° point while squeezing your shoulder bones together. Do 12-15 reps.

<u>4. Hip flexor stretch – extends the front of the hips</u>

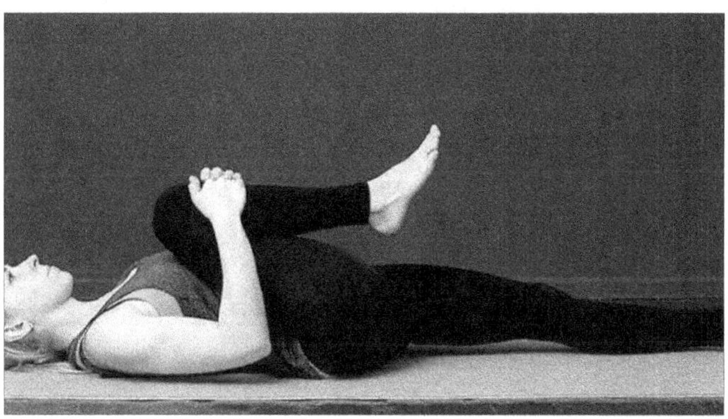

The most effective method to do it: get in a bowing position, propel yourself forward so your front knee starts to curve and you feel a stretch in the front region of the back leg. Hold for 15-30 seconds each side and repeat twice.

<u>5. Extension – enacts the glutes and center</u>

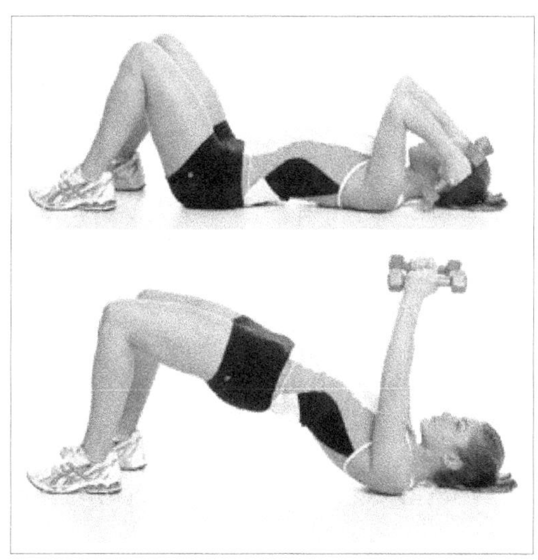

The most effective method to do it: set down on your back with your knees twisted. Press your glutes together, push through your heels, so your pelvis brings up noticeable all around. Pushing through your heels is critical to enact the glutes. Do 12-15 reps twice.

6. Youngster's posture – stretches the lower back

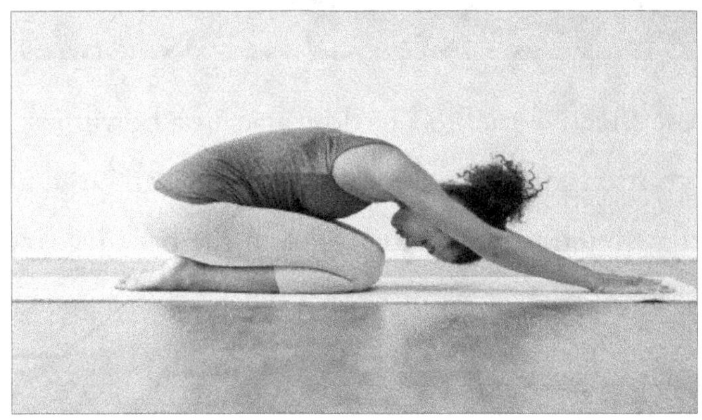

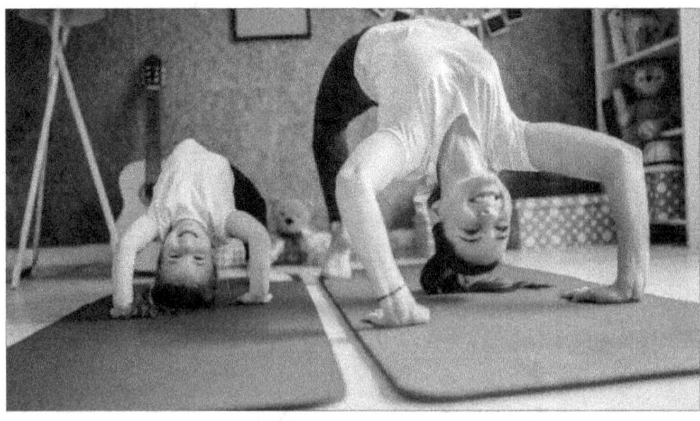

Step by step instructions to do it: sit on your knees, place your arms before your body on the floor, sit back towards your heels until you feel your back stretch. Hold for 15-30 seconds, repeat twice.

Exercise toward the end of the workday

It may be tempting to avoid any exercises in the wake of a monotonous day's worth of effort, and believe it or not, I don't blame you. 76% of laborers in the US feel tired many days during the week, leaving no inspiration to exercise.

What many people don't recognize is that even two or three minutes of exercise can significantly change your state of mind from slow and tired to stimulated and strengthened, diminishing exhaustion by as much as 65%.

When is the perfect time of day to work out?

Attempting to locate the best time for exercise? It's close to home! Follow these tips to make sense of what wellness routine works best for you.

First light, nightfall, or dead of night—when's the best time to work out? Indeed, that depends upon when's the best time for you, because the advantages of physical activity depend on how predictable you are.

You possibly have heard that the best time to exercise is toward the beginning of the day — to get your digestion moving or to keep away from sudden interruptions during the day that could crash your workout. Be that as it may, if you're not a morning individual, it may not work for you to attempt to find a workable pace to work out. The key is to do what's destined to work for you reliably.

If your calendar isn't rigid, you may be adaptable and have an arrangement for different times of day.

If you find that working out past the point of no return at night shields you from nodding off effectively, shift your exercise meeting prior in the day or attempt less exceptional, increasingly particular types of development.

CHAPTER 8

WHAT MAY BE MORE IMPORTANT, AND WHY?

To remain committed, pick exercises you appreciate. If you're a social individual, do something that connects with you socially. Take a group exercise class, join a recreational group, or take a stroll with a group of coworkers. If you are inclined toward having time alone, walking, swimming, or biking solo may be a better fit for you. If you'd prefer to invest more energy with your family, discover an activity you would all be able to do together, such as an after-supper walk or a round of soccer.

There are such a large number of decisions; don't restrict yourself to only one. Having an assortment of wellness exercises to browse may shield you from getting exhausted or worn out.

Below are a few exercises you can do anytime of the day:

- ❖ Walking, jogging and running

- ❖ Swimming

- ❖ Biking

- ❖ Moving and vigorous exercise

- ❖ Climbing stairs

- ❖ Playing sports

- ❖ Quality preparing and weights

- ❖ Yoga and pilates

- ❖ Boxing and kickboxing

- ❖ Hand to hand fighting and Tai Chi

There's no ideal time of day to get going. So do it at the time that is directly for you.

CHAPTER 9

STRETCHING AFTER EXERCISE ISN'T REALLY DOING WHAT YOU BELIEVE IT'S DOING?

There is a ton of debate concerning the worth or deficiency of muscle stretching to accelerate recovery after exercise. "Stretching gets out your lactic corrosive" and other comparable cases flourish. Is any of this genuine?

To start with, it is not easy to explain the difference between stretching for remodeling and stretching for recovery.

Recovery

Muscles are called upon to work during exercise. During this work, fuel is spent, squander items are made, and the muscle fiber structure is disturbed by numerous small scale tears. Envision a feast, for examination, during which the nourishment is eaten, trash is aggregated (napkins, chicken bones, and so forth), and the table settings upset. Before the following feast, the nourishment should be restocked, the trash cleared, and the tables reset.

For muscles, this procedure of resetting for the following event is called recovery. The muscle comes back to full capacity without irritation.

This isn't the procedure that prompts body change essentially. Yet, it is significant for competitors who wish to contend at their most elevated level on numerous occasions during a brief period.

Competitors have attempted numerous things to accelerate recovery: cryotherapy, rub, pressure, ice water drenching, stretching, hyperbaric oxygen, and hostile to inflammatories, to give some examples. These interventions are planned for diminishing lactic corrosive, incendiary markers, and different resorts that develop following extreme exercise.

Of these, the lone back rub is reliably compelling. Various studies have demonstrated that stretching doesn't help significantly in squander expulsion or serve in any way to accelerate muscle recovery.

Stretching After Exercise Isn't Really Doing What You Believe It's Doing?

<u>Remodeling</u>

A large portion of us aren't preparing for proficient rivalries but are wanting to be healthy, lose weight, and improve our temperaments.

For that, we have to concentrate on our body's remodeling response to exercise, which isn't equivalent to recovery from exercise.

Doubtlessly stated, when we exercise regularly, our bodies adjust to that stressor by changing our muscle structure, digestion, and physiology. It is that change, that remodeling, that prompts all the definite advantages of exercise. To stay with our meal model, if we understood that 500 individuals are going to appear at each event, yet we have ten tables set at present, we would change our ability to be prepared for the following event. We would expand the effectiveness in the kitchen and set more tables. In like manner, our body rebuilds itself to adjust to broadening exercise.

Numerous studies have been made showing how to streamline the body's remodeling response to exercise. Following 35 or more prolonged periods of study, six factors rise as reliably helping the body in its push to rearrange in response to exercise: timing of healthful admission (specifically protein), kind of exercise, knead, rest, low-portion creative and—you got it—stretching.

The most notable and acknowledged advantages of muscle stretching exercises are to improve or keep up the scope of movement, or both; the arrangement of bones and joints; and fortifying of connective tissues—all components that upgrade execution. Numerous studies have demonstrated that adaptability preparing (devoted consideration after some time to muscle stretching as a component of an exercise program) straightforwardly improves muscle capacity, and ultrasound pictures have recorded suitable adjustments in muscle design following a long period of regular stretching, for example, longer filaments. Also, an ongoing report has unmistakably demonstrated that stretching after some time improves blood flow to the muscles during consequent exercise in animals.

Earlier negative analysis around muscle stretching might be misdirecting to the easygoing spectator. The facts confirm that studies have demonstrated static stretching schedules (reach, hold for 30 seconds, discharge, next stretch) preceding a workout or athletic event leads to a reduction in quality during that event and that stretching before an activity doesn't prevent injuries, as was thought for some time. However, these are unmistakable conditions that don't matter to the vast majority.

CHAPTER 10

SO DO I STRETCH OR NOT?

If you are a tip-top competitor attempting to diminish your chances of injury, increase quality, or accelerate muscle recovery directly before your next event—at that point, no.

If you are like most people—wanting to lose weight, be well, and improve your state of mind—stretching will assist with muscle remodeling, connective tissue reinforcing, scope of movement improvement, joint arrangement, and improved blood flow during exercise.

CHAPTER 11

WHAT ARE THE PERFECT STRETCHES FOR TIGHT HAMSTRINGS?

The hamstrings are entirely defenseless to injury, and individuals who take part in sports that include running or jumping are inclined to create tightness or injury in these muscles.

The hamstrings refer to three different muscles in the back of the thigh that runs from the hip to the knee. These muscle groups allow us to walk, run, and hop.

Since people utilize their hamstrings in ordinary activities, for example, strolling, it is essential to keep these muscles loose. Stretching will assist people with keeping away from strains and muscle tears.

This report will examine seven of the best hamstring stretches, when to utilize them, how frequently to use them, and the advantages of a hamstring stretch.

Seven best hamstring stretches

Hamstring stretches will help keep the muscles adaptable and versatile. These stretches ought not to cause pain. Just stretch until it is gentle to direct pressure. Flexibility will improve over time, and individuals should abstain from overstretching, as this can cause injury.

Utilize the following stretches to loosen muscle tightness in the hamstrings:

1. Lying hamstring stretch

Lie flat on either the floor or a mat with your legs completely stretched out.

To stretch your right leg, hold the rear of the right knee with two hands, pull the leg up toward the chest, and gradually fix the knee until it feels as if it is stretching.

Hold the stretch for 10–30 seconds.

2. Lying hamstring stretch utilizing a tie

Lie flat on either the floor or a mat with your legs completely stretched out.

To stretch the right leg, bend the right leg and spot the tie over the bundle of the right foot.

Hold the tie in both hands.

Keep the left leg stretched out on the floor with the foot flexed so as to push the thigh and calf toward the floor.

Gradually lift the right leg with the foot flexed. The right leg ought to have a slight bend in the knee, and the base of the foot should be parallel with the ceiling.

Gently pull the tie until there is a slight pressure in the hamstrings.

Hold the stretch for 10–30 seconds.

Repeat several times.

3. Lying hamstring stretch utilizing a wall

Locate an open entryway.

Lie flat on either the floor or a mat, with your back flat and your left leg completely stretched out on the floor. The left leg should go through the entryway.

Lean the right leg against the wall by the entryway.

Modify the separation between your body and the wall to accomplish a slight strain in the correct leg.

Hold the stretch for 10–30 seconds.

Repeat several times.

4. Sitting hamstring stretch

To stretch the right leg, sit on the floor with the left leg bowed at the knee with the foot facing the floor. This is known as the butterfly position.

Lift the right leg, keeping it marginally twisted at the knee.

Bend forward at the abdomen, making a point to keep your back straight.

Hold the stretch for 10–30 seconds.

Repeat a few times.

5. Sitting hamstring stretch using a chair

Sit with your back straight close to the edge of the chair.

Keep your feet flat on the floor.

To stretch the right leg, fix it with your heel on the floor and your toes pointing to the ceiling.

Bend forward at your hip and spot your hands on your left leg for support.

Ensure the spine is in a neutral position.

Hold the stretch for 10–30 seconds.

Repeat several times.

6. <u>Standing hamstring stretch</u>

Stand upright with your spine in an unbiased position.

Spot the right leg in front of your body with your foot flexed, the heel in the floor and the toe pointing to the ceiling.

Bend your left knee somewhat.

Tenderly lean forward and place the hands on the straight right leg.

Keep a neutral spine.

Hold the stretch for 10–30 seconds.

Repeat several times.

7. Standing hamstring stretch utilizing a table

Locate a table that is shorter than the height of your hip.

Stand upright with your spine in an unbiased position.

Spot your right leg on the table with the foot flexed, so the toes point to the ceiling. Stand far enough away from the table with the goal that only your foot and part of the calf are on the table.

Bend forward at the midsection until there is a stretch in the hamstring muscle.

To increase the force of the stretch, bend forward somewhat, placing your hands on the leg or the table for help.

Hold up 15 seconds and repeat several times.

Your protection is essential to us.

Advantages of hamstring stretches

Hamstring stretches can keep the hamstrings adaptable and loose. Adaptable hamstrings have numerous advantages, for example:

What Are The Perfect Stretches For Tight Hamstrings?

Forestalling lower back pain

Tight hamstrings diminish the portability of the pelvis, which can squeeze the lower back. Reinforcing and stretching the hamstrings can keep them from getting excessively tight and offer additional help for the return and pelvis.

Decreasing wounds

Keeping the hamstrings loose will reduce the opportunity of stressing or tearing the muscle filaments during strenuous physical exercises, for example, running.

Expanding flexibility

Hamstring stretches can enhance flexibility and boost the scope of movement in the hip. Both of these advantages will assist individuals with performing day by day errands, for example, strolling upstairs and bending over, effortlessly.

Improving stance

At the point when the hamstrings are excessively tight, the muscles pivot the pelvis in reverse. This can flatten the characteristic curve in the back, which can cause weakness and standing stance. Keeping the hamstrings loose can assist individuals with sitting straighter and standing taller.

When to utilize hamstring stretches

- ❖ Individuals should stretch the muscles in their bodies, including the hamstrings, day by day. Indeed, even a couple of moments of daily stretching can improve an individual's general portability.

- ❖ If somebody encounters enduring tightness in their hamstrings, they ought to think about addressing their human services supplier. Steady tightness in the hamstrings may suggest that the muscles are over-lengthened.

- ❖ In these cases, stretching won't help, and the individual ought to instead concentrate on reinforcing their hamstrings.

- ❖ While the advantages of stretching when exercises are questionable, stretching is useful for in general wellbeing, as it improves flexibility and forestalls injury.

- ❖ Stretching the hamstrings will assist in keeping these muscles loose and adaptable, which will improve the act, increase flexibility, and forestall lower back agony.

CHAPTER 12

SIMPLE STRETCHES FOR KIDS

Straightforward stretches ought to be a standard part of children's physical activity schedule. Before or after a game practice or a long bicycle ride, before bed, or whenever your youngster's muscles feel tense or tight, urge them to attempt some simple stretches. They should stretch only when their muscles are heated up. So if they haven't recently been working out, they need to do a short warm-up, for example, moving or strolling or running set up.

The accompanying stretches for kids don't need to be done in a specific order. Yet, big or small, it is a smart idea to stretch the spine first and afterward move from the upper to the lower body. Hold each stretch for 20 to 30 seconds at the purpose of pressure or tightness—not pain—and repeat several times (switching legs and arms). Take your time in your stretch, and remember to relax.

If your youngster has a physical issue or is preparing for a specific game, counsel a physical advisor or athletic coach to decide the most secure and best approaches to stretching.

This appropriately named yoga present (called balasana in Sanskrit) is a decent route for children to start as well as end a stretching meeting. It's extremely unwinding!

Bend with toes contacting and knees spread separated. (A few people like to keep knees together. Attempt the two different ways to see which is increasingly agreeable.) Slowly twist around and contact the brow to the floor. Arms can be at the sides, palms facing up or stretched out before the head with palms on the floor. Breathe in and breathe out slowly; hold for 3 to 5 breaths.

Cat-cow

This yoga-affected stretch is useful for the spine and reinforces the muscular strength. Start down on the floor with the spine and neck in a neutral position. The back ought to be level like a tabletop. Eyes should look straight to the floor. Breathe in, drop the gut down, and gradually lift the neck and head up.

Next, on a breath out, lift the tummy and spine so the back is curved like a cat's. Eyes look toward the belly button.

Do 5 to 10 cat-cow stretches and come back to the neutral hands-and-knees position.

Overhead Arm Stretch

This basic yet viable stretch works the upper body, shoulders, and arms. Stand up straight with your feet together. With back straight, arrive at arms straight up and overhead, without locking elbows.

Hands can be contacting or separated. You can likewise do an exceptionally gentle backbend here. If you decide to twist backward, keep your jaw and neck lifted.

Arms Wide

This activity works with the arm and shoulder muscles. Remain with arms outstretched and thumbs pointing down. Gently push arms back as though pressing a ball between the shoulder bones.

On the other hand, gradually pivot the arms with the goal that thumbs are facing up. Hold and then pivot back to the principal position. Hold once more, gently pressing your arms again. Repeat a couple of times, continually moving gradually.

Shoulder Stretch

Arrive at the correct arm straight out before you. Curve the left-wing and put the left wrist on the back of the right arm, simply over the elbow. Your left palm will confront the side. Use the left arm to gently press the correct arm over your body until you feel a decent stretch. Hold for 10 to 30 seconds— switch arms and repeat.

Tricep Stretch

This stretch works the muscle on the rear of the upper arm. Raise the right arm up overhead, palm glancing in towards your head. At that point, twist the elbow so your fingers contact, or reach toward, the center of your upper back. Get the correct elbow with the left hand and gently pull back until you feel the stretch in the privilege tricep. Hold for 10 to 30 seconds. At that point, switch arms and repeat.

Knee Lunge

This may appear to be a leg stretch, yet it really works the muscles in the crotch. Start by bowing on a mat or delicate surface. Keeping your back straight, position your left foot on the ground, and gently press forward until the knee is twisted at a 90-degree angle (knee legitimately over the lower leg). This stretches the left hip and crotch.

Spot hands or elbows on the left knee to settle and hold for 10 to 30 seconds, without bobbing. Switch legs and repeat.

Butterfly Stretch

Children usually are very proficient at the butterfly stretch, which works the inward thighs and echoes the bungle present they may sit in whenever they're on the floor. This is sometimes known as the lotus position—although a good lotus present requires the feet and lower legs to lay on the thighs, which is exceptionally testing.

In a seated position, place the bottoms of the feet together and hold them with both hands. The legs are currently shaping the butterfly "wings". Elbows can be between the legs or lying on the knees. Gently press the knees down to extend the stretch. To include a spine stretch, twist forward from the upper back and arrive at brow toward feet.

Straddle Stretch

Sit on the floor or a mat with legs separated. The width of the straddle is up to you—whatever feels great and a touch of testing, without bringing on any pain.

When seated, twist gradually over the right leg, to the middle, and over the left leg. Hold each position for 10 to 30 seconds without bobbing. These stretches work the lower back, inward thighs, and hamstrings.

Quadricep Stretch

This move stretches the large muscles on the front of the thighs that we use for running. Stand against the back of a seat (a wall or a tree also works; you simply need support for balance). With the left arm on the chair, twist your right leg and lift it with your right hand. Gently press your foot toward your body until you feel the stretch in the front of the thigh. Hold for 10 to 30 seconds and switch legs.

You can also do this stretch with your opposite arm holding the foot. It is marginally all the more trying to adjust along these lines, but having a seat makes a difference.

Calf Stretch

Spot your forearms on a wall. Remain with one leg close to the wall. Broaden the other leg back, keeping the heel on the floor until you feel the stretch in the lower leg muscle (back of the lower leg). Hold for 10 to 30 seconds without bobbing.

Switch sides and repeat on the other leg. This stretch feels excellent after running or strolling.

Side Lunge

This stretch works the internal thighs, also called the adductors, and the hips. Stand up straight with legs separated, more extensive than hip separation. Twist one leg to a 90-degree angle and keep the other leg stretched out straight with toes and heels pointing at a 45-degree angle. Feel the stretch in the inward thigh and hold for 10 to 30 seconds. Hold back straight.

Switch sides and repeat.

Hybrid Toe Touch

Stretch the back and the hamstrings with a toe contact. Remain with arms hanging freely at sides and feet together, with knees marginally bowed. Gradually move down from the back and reach toward the toes with your hands. Contacting them is discretionary! Hold the stretch without skipping.

For a variety, fold the legs while standing. You can likewise chip away at toe contacts in a seated position. Continuously keep a slight twist in the knees. Keep in mind, not every person can contact their toes. Simply reach the extent that you can without pain. A little distress or pressure is alright.

Hamstring Stretch

In a seated position, extend the left leg straight forward, toes facing up. Twist your right leg and spot the bottom of the right foot along with the knee or internal thigh of the left leg. Reach forward toward the toes of your left foot until you experience the hamstring stretch. Hold for 10 to 30 seconds without bobbing.

Switch legs and repeat. This stretch is sometimes considered a hurdler's stretch since it copies the position of a sprinter's legs as they jump over obstacles.

CONCLUSION

<u>Stretching basics</u>

Before you dive into stretching, make sure you do it safely and successfully. While you can stretch anywhere and anytime, an appropriate method is vital. Improper stretching can cause more damage than good.

Utilize these tips to protect stretching:

* Try not to consider stretching a warm-up. You may hurt yourself if you stretch damaged muscles. Before stretching, warm up with light strolling, running, or biking at a low intensity for five to 10 minutes. Even better, stretch after your exercise when your muscles are warm.

* Consider skipping stretching before an extreme event, for example, dashing or Olympic style events exercises. Some research recommends that pre-event stretching may diminish execution. Research has likewise

demonstrated that stretching preceding an event debilitates hamstring quality.

❖ Additionally, take a stab at playing out a "dynamic warm-up". A dynamic warm-up includes performing activities like those in your sport or physical movement at a low level and slowly increasing speed and intensity as you warm up.

❖ Take a stab at balance. Everybody's hereditary qualities for flexibility are somewhat different. As opposed to making progress toward the flexibility of an artist or athlete, focus on having equivalent flexibility on both sides (particularly if you have experienced a past injury). The flexibility that isn't equivalent to both sides might be a precursor for injury.

❖ Focus your stretches on major muscle groups, for example, your calves, thighs, hips, lower back, neck, and shoulders. Make sure that you stretch both sides.

❖ Additionally, stretch muscles and joints that you routinely use.

❖ Try not to rebound. Stretch in a smooth motion without skipping. Ricocheting as you stretch can harm your muscles and add to muscle tightness.

* Hold your stretch. Inhale and hold each stretch for around 30 seconds; in some areas, you may need to hold for around 60 seconds.

* Try not to focus on the pain. Hope to feel strain while you're stretching, not pain. If it harms you, you've gone too far. Chill out to where you don't feel any pain. At that point, hold the stretch.

* Make stretches sport-specific. Some studies suggest that it's useful to do stretches for the muscles used most in your sport or activity. If you play soccer, for instance, stretch your hamstrings as you're increasingly defenseless against hamstring strains.

* Stay aware of your stretching. Stretching can be tedious. In any case, you can accomplish the most advantages by stretching routinely, for example, a few times each week.

* Avoiding regular stretching causes you to risk losing the potential advantages. For instance, if stretching helped you increase your scope of movement, your range of motion may diminish again if you quit stretching.

* Bring development into your stretching. Gentle events, for example, those in kendo or yoga, can assist you with being progressively adaptable in specific developments.

These sorts of activities can likewise help you get more established with other stretching.

* ❖ Remember the "dynamic warm-up": If you play out a specific action, for example, a kick in combative techniques or kicking a soccer ball, begin slowly and at a low intensity to get your muscles accustomed to it, then continuously speed up.

Realize when to practice alertness

If you have a chronic condition or an injury, you may need to modify your stretching strategies. For instance, if you have a strained muscle, stretching it might bring on additional harm. Consult with your primary care physician or physical specialist about the most suitable approach to stretch if you have any health concerns.

The End

Thanks for taking the time to read my book. I hope it helped you out in some type of way. If you are not already please go now and follow me here on FB here

https://www.facebook.com/RichardRobertson40/ or here https://www.instagram.com/stayingfitafter40club on instagram .

By following me you will receive updates on all of my upcoming books, giveaways, also you will be the first to get free copies of all of my books.

Never miss another update

You can also follow me here on my Author's Page on Amazon.

Just Because

Just because you took the time to read my book here are two of my Books **FREE**. Sign up and get your books.

The guide to staying healthy after 40 for women...The Keto way

&

Staying fit after 40